PERFUME

The complete Guide To Create Your own

Natural Scent Signature

By Ori Laor

Disclaimer

The methods described within this eBook are the author's personal thoughts. They are not intended to be a definitive set of instructions for this project. You may discover there are other methods and materials to accomplish the same end result.

This book is not intended to be a substitute for the medical advice of a licensed physician. The reader should consult with their doctor in any matters relating to his/her health.

Before beginning any new exercise program, it is recommended that you seek medical advice from your personal physician.

The information contained within this eBook is strictly for educational purposes. If you wish to apply ideas contained in this eBook, you are taking full responsibility for your actions.

The author has made every effort to ensure the accuracy of the information within this book was correct at time of publication. The author does not assume and hereby disclaims any liability to any party for any loss, damage, or disruption caused by errors or omissions, whether such errors or omissions result from accident, negligence, or any other cause.

Thank you very much
Ori Laor

Table of Contents

Personal Introduction

Thank you for downloading this fantastic guide - "PERFUME - The complete Guide To Create Your own Natural Scent Signature". I am a perfume creator for many years, helping people create theire own scent signature in this world. I have created this book for any one who wants to be special and understand the world of Perfume.

The word perfume derives from the Latin "per fumum", meaning through smoke. Perfumery, or the art of making perfumes, began in ancient Mesopotamia and Egypt and was further refined by the Romans and Persians. Knowledge of perfumery came to Europe as early as the 14th century due partially to the spread of Islam.

The first modern perfume, made of scented oils blended in an alcohol solution, was made in 1370 at the command of Queen Elizabeth of Hungary and was known throughout Europe as Hungary Water. The art of perfumery prospered in Renaissance Italy, and in the 16th century, Italian refinements were taken to France by Catherine de' Medici's personal perfumer, Rene le Florentin. His laboratory was connected with her apartments by a secret passageway, so that no formulas could be stolen en route.

France quickly became the European center of perfume and cosmetic manufacture. Cultivation of flowers for their perfume essence, which had begun in the 14th century, grew into a major industry in the south of France. During the Renaissance period, perfumes were used primarily by the wealthy to mask body odors resulting from infrequent bathing. Partly due to this patronage, the western perfumery industry was created. By the 18th century, aromatic plants were being grown in the Grasse region of France to provide the growing perfume industry with raw materials. Even today, France remains the centre of the European perfume design and trade.

Why is it that women love perfume as much as men love cars? There are some researchers who believe that a woman's reason for loving perfume is because of the pheromones their bodies produce. Often, certain scents or perfumes trigger the increase of how much pheromone a woman's body will produce. While a perfume will help in increasing the production of a woman's pheromone levels, they are also liked by women because of the attention they get from a member of the opposite sex or even from another woman. In studies carried out, nearly 80% of all women will make a perfume purchase at least once each year.

Many women will tell you that the reason they purchase a particular perfume for themselves is that it makes them smell great and they seem to feel better about themselves. It also makes them feel a little bit more feminine. Not only does smelling great make a woman feel good about herself, but it will make her feel attractive also. In this book, a personal guide to create the perfect smell signature, and unlike any of those that you can buy either in store or over the internet.

Perfume is a combination of a secret chemistry between the heart and the soul. It can make us feel good or bad smell can leave us badly heart. All my life I looked for the perfect scent and over the years I noticed that the taste is changing and new opportunities of scents are open all the time.

In This book, I will take your hand and guide you throw everything you need to do to create your own Perfume. I will help you make natural scents that will feet you like a glove and will turn the heads of every one.

For my new Kindle readers, I offer a Free Voucher Gift of 20$. You can find a keyword at the end of this book. Please send it to my mail orilaor@outlook.com, and you will receive a discount for any porches you make for yourself, a member of your family or a friend in LAOR website www.laorcare.com.

About Me

I have a passion for Beauty, Skincare, Anti-aging and well-being methods. In my extensive exploration around the world, I gathered sacred pieces of information that helped me and then other people from all walks of life to look and feel younger. I hold a BA in Art and diplomas for Makeup Artist, Para Medical Aesthetician, Aromatherapy, Naturopathy, and Nutrition consultant. I am a well-known name in T.V scene and in the cosmetic industry, including treating many celebrities. When I was 30 years old, I quit working for others and founded LAOR, a House of natural Beauty and Professional Skin Care and treatments for the face, Body, and Mind.

Since an early age, I suffered from my skin and was carried away with Skincare research, science and well-being. I worked in beauty and style departments in New York and Tel Aviv, based on my experience I invented a revolutionary practice for treating the skin from within – **The Layer system**, Complied with a line of professional cosmetic products and treatments for the face to treat any skin problem.

Ientered the natural cosmetics world with a unique world-view and with one simple, honest purpose: to create a different kind of cosmetic that is Natural and effective. My desire is that each product would provide each with the essence of beauty, based on effective ingredients.

Now, for the past Two Decades, I am designing the products that Men and women across the world love, helping them to look and feel younger with all the secrets of skin care. When I am not working, I love to design and create, read, write and paint. My quest is to bring more beauty to the world and raise self-awareness.

Let's Get Started!

Chapter 1

Aromatherapy

Aromatherapy uses plant materials and aromatic plant oils, including essential oils, and other aroma compounds for improving psychological or physical well-being.It can be offered as a complementary therapy or, more controversially, as a form of alternative medicine. Complementary therapy can be offered alongside standard treatment, with alternative medicine offered instead of conventional, evidence-based treatments. Aromatherapists, who specialize in the practice of aromatherapy, utilize blends of therapeutic essential oils that can be issued through topical application, massage, inhalation or water immersion to stimulate a desired response.There is no good medical evidence that aromatherapy can either prevent or cure any disease, but it might help improve general well-being.

Aromatherapy is the practice of using volatile plant oils, including essential oils, for psychological and physical well-being.Essential oils, the pure essence of a plant, have been found to provide both psychological and physical benefits when used correctly and safely. The Essential Oil Profiles area details over 90 essential oils. Absolutes, CO2s and Hydrosols are also commonly utilized in aromatherapy. Although essential oils, CO2 extracts and absolutes are distilled by different methods, the term essential oil is sometimes used as a blanket term to include all natural, aromatic, volatile, plant oils including CO2s and absolutes.

In addition to essential oils, aromatherapy encourages the use of other complementary natural ingredients including cold pressed vegetable oils, jojoba (a liquid wax), hydrosols, herbs, milk powders, sea salts, sugars (an exfoliant), clays and muds. Products that include synthetic ingredients are frowned upon in holistic aromatherapy. It is important to note that perfume oils also known as fragrance oils (and usually listed as "fragrance" on an ingredient label) are not the same as essential oils. Fragrance oils and perfume oils contain synthetic chemicals and do not provide the therapeutic benefits of essential oils.

Aromatherapy Works

A common question that people ask when they first meet an aromatherapist is, 'how does aromatherapy work?' Good question. From the very start of aromatherapy's resurgence back in the 1980's, how aromatherapy works together with essential oils has been a somewhat misunderstood subject. Well, the name is a bit misleading since there is far more to it than just smelling aromas. Hardly surprising it was met with ridicule for the first 10 years! So here are some of the most important facts about the way that aromatherapy helps improve your health and well being. When essential oils are applied to the body they penetrate the skin via the hair follicles and sweat glands and are absorbed into the body fluids, where they not only help to kill bacteria and viruses but also stimulate the body's immune system, thereby strengthening resistance to further attack.

Some essential oils increase the circulation and help with the efficient elimination of toxins, others promote new cell growth and encourage the body's natural ability to heal itself. Each essential oil has its own character and aroma, exhibiting a varying number of properties and benefits which are unique to itself, since no two essential oils are quite the same. The minute molecules of essential oils are readily absorbed into the bloodstream when they are inhaled as the lungs work to oxygenate the blood. This form of absorption is most efficient when inhaling essential oils from a tissue, diffusing them in a vaporizer, or adding them to your bathwater. The aroma sends a signal directly to the Limbic System in the brain which is the centre of emotions, memory and sexual arousal. This is why essential oils have such a powerful effect on our moods and general state of mind.

We like all animals react to smells and the chemistry between people is built on the basic of personal scents.

Chapter 2

The Basic Perfume Pallet

Fragrance 'Notes'

Are the ingredients used to make up the perfume, and can range from plant and flower extracts to synthetically-created molecules. New technology can recreate the essence of almost any scent on earth, with recent examples including candy floss, sea salt and caramel. What do the 'Top', 'Heart' and 'Base' categories mean?

Top Notes: Top notes are evident as soon as the liquid touches your skin. These are usually lighter than the other ingredients, and function by shaping the primary fragrance burst.

Heart or Middle Notes: Shortly after application, the top notes give way to the heart notes. These are usually floral, as most fruity notes are too light for this layer. These middle notes make up the core perfume as it sits on the skin, and it is these layers that define the ultimate dry down, when the perfume settles on to the skin.

Base notes: The base notes determine how long a fragrance will last, and provide a background on which the heart notes can be appreciated. Interestingly, most fragrances have similar base notes, often including sandalwood, amber, musk and vanilla. This is because there are only a certain number of notes that will last long enough on the skin to form the base of a fragrance.

How it is built from mostly natural ingredients

According to the Bible, Three Wise Men visited the baby Jesus carrying myrrh and frankincense. Ancient Egyptians burned incense called kyphi made of henna, myrrh, cinnamon, and juniper as religious offerings. They soaked aromatic wood, gum, and resins in water and oil and used the liquid as a fragrant body lotion. The early Egyptians also perfumed their dead and often assigned specific fragrances to deities.

Their word for perfume has been translated as "fragrance of the gods." It is said that the Moslem prophet Mohammed wrote, "Perfumes are foods that reawaken the spirit." Eventually Egyptian perfumery influenced the Greeks and the Romans. For hundreds of years after the fall of Rome, perfume was primarily an Oriental art. It spread to Europe when 13th century Crusaders brought back samples from Palestine to England, France, and Italy. Europeans discovered the healing properties of fragrance during the 17th century. Doctors treating plague victims covered their mouths and noses with leather pouches holding pungent cloves, cinnamon, and spices which they thought would protect them from disease. Perfume then came into widespread use among the monarchy. France's King Louis XIV used it so much that he was called the "perfume king." His court contained a floral pavilion filled with fragrances, and dried flowers were placed in bowls throughout the palace to freshen the air. Royal guests bathed in goat's milk and rose petals. Visitors were often doused with perfume, which also was sprayed on clothing, furniture, walls, and tableware. It was at this time that Grasse, a region of southern France where many flowering plant varieties grow, became a leading producer of perfumes.

Meanwhile, in England, aromatics were contained in lockets and the hollow heads of canes to be sniffed by the owner. It was not until the late 1800s, when synthetic chemicals were used, that perfumes could be mass marketed. The first synthetic perfume was nitrobenzene, made from nitric acid and benzene. This synthetic mixture gave off an almond smell and was often used to scent soaps. In 1868, Englishman

William Perkin synthesized coumarin from the South American tonka bean to create a fragrance that smelled like freshly sown hay. Ferdinand Tiemann of the University of Berlin created synthetic violet and vanilla. In the United States, Francis Despard Dodge created citronellol — an alcohol with rose-like odor — by experimenting with citronella, which is derived from citronella oil and has a lemon-like odor. In different variations, this synthetic compound gives off the scents of sweet pea, lily of the valley, narcissus, and hyacinth.

Just as the art of perfumery progressed through the centuries, so did the art of the perfume bottle. Perfume bottles were often as elaborate and exotic as the oils they contained. The earliest specimens date back to about 1000 B.C. In ancient Egypt, newly invented glass bottles were made largely to hold perfumes. The crafting of perfume bottles spread into Europe and reached its peak in Venice in the 18th century, when glass containers assumed the shape of small animals or had pastoral scenes painted on them. Today perfume bottles are designed by the manufacturer to reflect the character of the fragrance inside, whether light and flowery or dark and musky.

The Raw Materials

Natural ingredients flowers, grasses, spices, fruit, wood, roots, resins, balsams, leaves, gums, and animal secretions as well as resources like alcohol, petrochemicals, coal, and coal tars are used in the manufacture of perfumes. Some plants, such as lily of the valley, do not produce oils naturally. In fact, only about 2,000 of the 250,000 known flowering plant species contain these essential oils. Therefore, synthetic chemicals must be used to re-create the smells of non-oily substances. Synthetics also create original scents not found in nature. Some perfume ingredients are animal products. For example, castor comes from beavers, musk from male deer, and ambergris from the sperm whale. Animal substances are often used as fixatives that enable perfume to evaporate slowly and emit odors longer. Other fixatives include coal tar, mosses, resins, or synthetic chemicals. Alcohol and sometimes water are used to dilute ingredients in perfumes. It is the ratio of alcohol to scent that determines whether the perfume is "eau de toilette" (toilet water) or cologne.

Manufacturing Process

Extraction - Oils are extracted from plant substances by several methods: steam distillation, solvent extraction, enfleurage, maceration, and expression.

1. Before the manufacturing process begins, the initial ingredients must be brought to the manufacturing center. Plant substances are harvested from around the world, often hand-picked for their fragrance. Animal products are obtained by extracting the fatty substances directly from the animal. Aromatic chemicals used in synthetic perfumes are created in the laboratory by perfume chemists.

2. In steam distillation, steam is passed through plant material held in a still, whereby the essential oil turns to gas. This gas is then passed through tubes, cooled, and liquified. Oils can also be extracted by boiling plant substances like flower petals in water instead of steaming them.

3. Under solvent extraction, flowers are put into large rotating tanks or drums and benzene or a petroleum ether is poured over the flowers, extracting the essential oils. The flower parts dissolve in the solvents

and leave a waxy material that contains the oil, which is then placed in ethyl alcohol. The oil dissolves in the alcohol and rises. Heat is used to evaporate the alcohol, which once fully burned off, leaves a higher concentration of the perfume oil on the bottom. Oils are extracted from plant substances by steam disfillation, solvent extraction, enfleurage, maceration, or expression.

4. During enfleurage, flowers are spread on glass sheets coated with grease. The glass sheets are placed between wooden frames in tiers. Then the flowers are removed by hand and changed until the grease has absorbed their fragrance.

5. Maceration is similar to enfleurage except that warmed fats are used to soak up the flower smell. As in solvent extraction, the grease and fats are dissolved in alcohol to obtain the essential oils.

6. Expression is the oldest and least complex method of extraction. By this process, now used in obtaining citrus oils from the rind, the fruit or plant is manually or mechanically pressed until all the oil is squeezed out.

7. Once the perfume oils are collected, they are ready to be blended together according to a formula determined by a master in the field, known as a "nose." It may take as many as 800 different ingredients and several years to develop the special formula for a scent.

After the scent has been created, it is mixed with alcohol. The amount of alcohol in a scent can vary greatly. Most full perfumes are made of about 10-20% perfume oils dissolved in alcohol and a trace of water. Colognes contain approximately 3-5% oil diluted in 80-90% alcohol, with water making up about 10%. Toilet water has the least amount—2% oil in 60-80% alcohol and 20% water.

Aging - Fine perfume is often aged for several months or even years after it is blended. Following this, a "nose" will once again test the perfume to ensure that the correct scent has been achieved. Each essential oil and perfume has three notes: "Notes de tete," or top notes, "notes de coeur," central or heart notes, and "notes de fond," base notes. Top notes have tangy or citrus-like smells; central notes (aromatic flowers like rose and jasmine) provide body, and base notes (woody fragrances) provide an enduring fragrance. More "notes," of various smells, may be further blended.

Quality Control - Because perfumes depend heavily on harvests of plant substances and the availability of animal products, perfumery can often turn risky. Thousands of flowers are needed to obtain just one pound of essential oils, and if the season's crop is destroyed by disease or adverse weather, perfumeries could be in jeopardy. In addition, consistency is hard to maintain in natural oils. The same species of plant raised in several different areas with slightly different growing conditions may not yield oils with exactly the same scent.

Problems are also encountered in collecting natural animal oils. Many animals once killed for the value of their oils are on the endangered species list and now cannot be hunted. For example, sperm whale products like ambergris have been outlawed since 1977. Also, most animal oils in general are difficult and expensive to extract. Deer musk must come from deer found in Tibet and China; civet cats, bred in Ethiopia, are kept for their fatty gland secretions; beavers from Canada and the former Soviet Union are harvested for their castor. Synthetic perfumes have allowed perfumers more freedom and stability in their craft, even though natural ingredients are considered more desirable in the very finest perfumes. The use of synthetic perfumes and oils eliminates the need to extract oils from animals and removes the risk of a bad plant harvest, saving much expense and the lives of many animals.

The Future Of Perfume

Perfumes today are being made and used in different ways than in previous centuries. Perfumes are being manufactured more and more frequently with synthetic chemicals rather than natural oils. Less concentrated forms of perfume are also becoming increasingly popular. Combined, these factors decrease the cost of the scents, encouraging more widespread and frequent, often daily, use. Using perfume to heal, make people feel good, and improve relationships between the sexes are the new frontiers being explored by the industry. The sense of smell is considered a right brain activity, which rules emotions, memory, and creativity. Aromatherapy smelling oils and fragrances to cure physical and emotional problems is being revived to help balance hormonal and body energy. The theory behind aromatherapy states that using essential oils helps bolster the immune system when inhaled or applied topically. Smelling sweet smells also affects one's mood and can be used as a form of psychotherapy.

Like aromatherapy, more research is being conducted to synthesize human perfume that is, the body scents we produce to attract or repel other humans. Humans, like other mammals, release pheromones to attract the opposite sex. New perfumes are being created to duplicate the effect of pheromones and stimulate sexual arousal receptors in the brain. Not only may the perfumes of the future help people cover up "bad" smells, they could improve their physical and emotional well-being as well as their sex lives.

The different kind of perfumes :

- ✓ Perfume

- ✓ Eau de perfume

- ✓ Eau de toilet

- ✓ Eau de cologne

What Are Fragrances?

Fragrances are complex mixtures of what people in the industry refer to as raw materials. These raw materials can be extracts from natural sources or synthetic raw materials. Oils are dissolved in a solvent (usually alcohol), to preserve a pleasant concoction of scents. The higher the concentration of oils – the greater the strength of the fragrance. The strength determines how long an application of the fragrance lasts on your skin. Fragrances come in many forms and have many different names but generally the main four categories are as follows:

Perfume: The perfume you see in the store is not the pure perfume essence and has been diluted. However it is the most concentrated of all the fragrance options and it is the most expensive for this reason. It tends to be slightly oilier and will typically contain 15-40% pure perfume extract. It has a slightly thicker, oilier consistency. It tends to be sold with 'stopper bottles' and not sprays. It is too strong to spray all over (and too expensive).

The percentage of pure perfume extract is not necessarily an indicator of the quality of perfume though. As mentioned there are many essential oils that you wouldn't want to smell like in small doses (spikenard comes to mind). Real musk and ambergris are expensive and not pleasant in their pure form, so whereas a single drop can dramatically increase the price of a perfume, but you wouldn't want more than that single drop, which would be sublime.

Eau de Perfume/(Parfum): This uses the same perfume essence but less of it and more alcohol and water. This means the smell is a bit lighter and usually doesn't last quite as long, but as it is a bit lighter, many find this preferable. It is of course cheaper. Typically there will be 10-20% perfume essence in Eau de Perfume. This perfume might be sold in normal bottles or sprays, but if a spray is used, it shouldn't be just doused all over.

Eau de Toilette: This is lighter still and usually sold in spray bottles. The lightness of it makes it more suitable to spray more liberally, the high alcohol content means it will not last very long. Generally this version is the most advisable to use day to day as it is less intense and even if you do use too much it will lighten up fairly quickly. Typically there will be 4-15% pure perfume essence.

Eau de Cologne: Cologne is an abbreviation of 'eau de Cologne' and is the French word for the city of Köln where a particular scent was first made hence it was a water from Cologne. There are specific blends of fragrances that fall in this particular category of 'eau de cologne', they are very light, fresh and fruity and contain the essential oils, lemon, bergamot, orange and also the absolute neroli. They may also contain the essential oils lavender and rosemary.

These days though, eau de cologne or cologne is also used to determine the most diluted version of the perfume. Typically 2-5%. These are rarely used in expensive perfumes, but tend to be more 'splash' kind of perfumes or fragrances for younger people.

Chapter 3

Choosing your Perfumes

Choosing your favorite scent is different from one to the other, everyone has its own taste and the combinations are endless. Choosing a perfume that is just right for you can feel like an overwhelming task. Given the thousands of fragrances on the market, it may seem easier just to stick with what you've always known. If that were the case for me, I'd still be wearing the 1986 version of Liz Claiborne perfume -- the one in the red triangle-shaped bottle. Overall, yes, it can be overwhelming to find the right fragrance. The perfume you wear is a personal choice; it's not like the clothes you borrow from your best friend. The fragrance your best friend wears might not work with your particular body chemistry. Besides, fragrance is a very personal choice. People will remember you for it. They will compliment you on it. They will ask what you're wearing. You'll wear it on first dates or for your wedding. If you arm yourself with proper knowledge, then shopping for the right fragrance won't be such a daunting task.

Fragrances are categorized according to notes, accords or other characteristics that define their overall similarities. More often than not, we tend to lean toward a particular fragrance family whether we know it or not.

Fragrance Families

Fresh: Fragrances categorized as fresh often include "green" notes, like fresh-cut grass, the smell of spring in the air, light citruses and airy notes. If you have an outdoorsy personality, a fragrance with fresh notes might be best for you.

Floral: Probably the most popular of all fragrance categories, floral scents encompass a wide range of blooms, from a single rose petal to a medley of floral bouquets. Floral scents may include notes of jasmine, carnation, gardenia, orange blossom, rose, lily of the valley, tuberose ... you name it. Floral scents can be powdery or sweet, depending on their combinations. If you enjoy the scent of a particular flower, maybe you should try fragrances that include notes of that flower.

Oriental: Just like its name suggests, the Oriental fragrance group is comprised of notes that are rich, bold and overall exotic. Notes like amber and vanilla are oftentimes present in the oriental group. Oriental fragrances lean toward the "heavier" side and are more sensual fragrances, ideal for nighttime wear or romantic occasions.

Woods (or Chypre): This fragrance group consists of your aromatic wood and moss notes -- sandalwood, cedarwood, oak. Patchouli is sometimes present, as is vetiver and pine. Many masculine fragrances fall into this category, given the richness of woody scents.

Fragrance Personality

Outdoorsy or sporty: If you live by a who-needs-makeup philosophy and your idea of weekend fun is camping in the great outdoors, you may prefer a fresh, citrus fragrance. Citrus fragrances are invigorating and light, unlike orientals which tend to command a room. Your personality type doesn't want the fragrance to stand out, rather complement your personality. You may lean toward unisex and green, herbacious fragrances as well.

Examples: Guerlain Eau de Guerlain, Chanel Cristalle, Eau de Cartier, Jo Malone Grapefruit, Dior Eau Savage, Yves Saint Laurent Y

Elegant: Maybe your weekends are lined up with black-tie dinner parties, and fragrance is much more than an afterthought. Oriental fragrances may be the best option for you. Rich and oppulent, these fragrances stand out and linger for hours. You may prefer a floral oriental (orange flower, vanilla) or a woody oriental (sandalwood, patchouli and spice).

Examples: Kenzo Flower, Guerlain L'Instant de Guerlain, Armani Code Pour Femme, Dolce & Gabbana the One, Yves Saint Laurent Opium, Shalimar by Guerlain, Calvin Klein Obsession

Girl-Next-Door: You have that certain Jennifer Aniston appeal; a little shy, a little sexy, but overall the girl he (or she) takes home to Mom. Fresh, clean scents are ideal as are woody florals. The latter might seem slightly more masculine, but woody notes can really bring out a shy girl's sex appeal.

Examples: Christian Dior's J'adore, Estee Lauder Pure White Linen, Victoria Secret's Very Sexy, Tom Ford Black Orchid, Calvin Klein Secret Obsession

All-American Guy - You're athletic, handsome and playful. Your fragrance must be able to stand up to the challenge, but not overwhelm the room. Fresh, water scents are great options, as are light woods.

Examples: Bvlgari Aqua, Lacoste Challenge, Davidoff Cool Water, Touch for Men by Burberry, L'Eau d'Issey Pour Homme, Clean Men by Dlish

Sophisticated, Modern Man: You keep up with the latest clothing trends and prefer your fitted trousers to Euro-shoes to jeans anyday. A touch of classic goes a long way. Fresh, crisp fragrances are perfect for you. Throw in some sweet florals and you've got a winner.

Examples: Acqua Di Gio Pour Homme by Giorgio Armani, Sean John Unforgivable, HM by Hanae Mori, Banana Republic Republic of Men.

You can buy in health shops or order on line from all over the world essential oil or fragrances as according to your personal taste. The most important thing is to love each scent individually, If you don't love it it is not for you !

The Classic Ones Are :

Top notes : Also called the head notes. The scents that are perceived immediately on application of a perfume. Top notes consist of small, light molecules that evaporate quickly. They form a person's initial impression of a perfume and thus are very important in the selling of a perfume. Examples of top notes are:

- ✓ Mint
- ✓ Cajuput
- ✓ Lavender
- ✓ Cinnamon
- ✓ coriander
- ✓ neroli
- ✓ Eucalyptus
- ✓ Lemon
- ✓ Mandarin /Tangerine
- ✓ orange
- ✓ Lime
- ✓ petit green
- ✓ grape fruit

Middle notes: Also referred to as heart notes. The scent of a perfume that emerges just prior to the dissipation of the top note. The middle note compounds form the "heart" or main body of a perfume and act to mask the often unpleasant initial impression of base notes, which become more pleasant with time. Examples of middle notes are:

- ✓ seawater,

- ✓ sandalwood

- ✓ Black Pepper

- ✓ Geranium

- ✓ Jasmin

- ✓ Spikenard

- ✓ Yarrow

- ✓ Nutmeg

- ✓ Palma Rosa

- ✓ Rosemary

- ✓ Lemon grass

- ✓ Ylang ylang

- ✓ Rosewood

- ✓ jasmine.

Base notes: The scent of a perfume that appears close to the departure of the middle notes. The base and middle notes together are the main theme of a perfume. Base notes bring depth and solidity to a perfume. Compounds of this class of scents are typically rich and "deep" and are usually not perceived until 30 minutes after application. Examples of base notes are:

- ✓ Benzoin
- ✓ Patchouli
- ✓ Balsam Peru
- ✓ Vanilla
- ✓ Vetiver
- ✓ Lavender
- ✓ Sandalwood
- ✓ Cassia
- ✓ Tobacco
- ✓ Clove
- ✓ Amber
- ✓ Myrrh
- ✓ Frankincense
- ✓ Musk.

The scents in the top and middle notes are influenced by the base notes, as well the scents of the base notes will be altered by the type of fragrance materials used as middle notes. Manufacturers of perfumes usually publish perfume notes and typically they present it as fragrance pyramid, with the components listed in imaginative and abstract terms.

Chapter 4

Anti-Aging Perfume

Some ingredients are considered for thousands of years to be the fountain of youth. This ingredients help our immune system and give us a wonderful uplifting feelings. Archaeologists discovered a perfume factory consisting of 43,000 square feet which is roughly the size of an acre of land. The 'factory' was filled with bottles, funnels, sixty stills dating 4000 years ago. In ancient times herbs and spices were used to produce perfume. Women and men have always relied on scent to distinguish themselves from others. Today, as it turns out, herbs and spices still play a role in perfumes and colognes along with flowers, leaves and twigs, fruits and seeds. Essentially anything organic may be considered as a base for perfume, including synthetic essences and essential oils.

Young Youthful Perfume

If you are trying to understand which perfumes have a youthful smell to them, knowing the basics is paramount. Below are 5 different standard categories all perfumes can be roughly divided into. This is a very simplistic list just for general reference, ingredients presented below can overlap into 2 or more categories:

Floral perfumes: jasmine, rose, gardenia

Oriental perfumes: sandalwood, patchouli, amber, musk

Woody perfumes: cedar, cinnamon

Fougère (Fern) perfumes: lavender, geranium, moss, wood

Fresh perfumes: citrus, grass, herbs, aquatics

Can a perfume actually perform a miracle and make one younger? No, of course not but a perfume can have an effect on the people who smell it permeating from your body hence producing a direct anti-aging effect. Odors have an effect on how we feel about ourselves and how others perceive us.

Pink Grapefruit – a smell of Youth

Scents that fall into the anti-aging perfume category are generally in line with the feminine notes of the last two groups: Fougère (lavender and geranium) and Fresh. Avoid all 'heavy, suffocating notes', as they are all scents that ooze maturity. Instead opt for lighter florals and citrus mixes. One study by the perfume house of Harvey Prince showed that women wearing scents with a blend of citrus and florals were perceived to be on average 6.7 years younger than their actual age. A later study showed the combination of mango and pink grapefruit was the olfactory (the perception of smells) antidote to aging as people were perceived as up to 12 years younger than their chronological age!

We have put together a list of 5 fragrances for you – all guaranteed to help you capture that youthful smell. The most important thing is how the fragrance interacts with your own chemistry so it is best to wear a sample for at least a day before buying.

1. Happy by Clinique

Fresh, clean scent with hints of ruby red grapefruit and plenty of light floral mixes to produce a perfume that can last all day without ever taking on any sour notes. The citrus fusion keeps it crisp, uplifting and – well, happy smelling!

2. Versense by Versace

Versense is a great example of an anti-aging perfume. It is considered fresh, luminous and sensual containing jasmine, rare flowers, sea lily, bergamot and zesty green mandarin.

3. Brit Sheer by Burberry

Once again this is a fresh, light but long lasting fragrance that packs a big punch as far as the right ingredients for an anti-aging perfume. There are hints of litchi, yuzu, pineapple leaf and mandarin orange as well as peony, peach blossom and pear; white musk and white woods... It is considered an energetic and adventurous mix.

4. Omnia Crystalline EDP by Bvlgari

This is a floral – light powdery scent with a hint of lotus, mandarin, iris root and sandalwood, Siam benzoin and musk. This is a young perfume as it has a light powdery but long lasting odor which reminds people of the femininity and everlasting beauty.

5. Warm Cotton (Reserve Blend) by Clean Reserve

Fresh, clean and not overly powdery but just perfect for those who are into soft florals. Romantic, cuddly and long lasting with strokes of Aldehydic Ginger, Watery Ozonic, Mint Green, Pepper Floral Accord, Musk, Incense and Vetiver. The ingredients again follow the path of nostalgic and comforting scents.

Mixing some rare essential oils in basic oils or butters can create the most amazing moisturizer working on the soul and the skin

Mixing Essential Oils

Mixing essential oils at home As I'm starting out, I'm thinking mixing essential oils is quite intimidating! How do I know how much to use of each oil? Which oils go together? What effect will the combined oils have? Will they complement each other and really make my aromatherapy recipes work? What I know so far, is that blending essential oils is definitely part art, and part science. Group your essential oils. Before beginning to create your own aromatherapy recipes of any sort, a good starting point is to categorize your essential oils into groups that share similar traits. This can be by what they do (effects you're after), how they smell (scent type), or if you want to be really technical, you'll sort them by their chemical make-up of how fast each of them evaporates (notes).

Grouping essential oils by the type of effects they have actually makes the most sense to me; I find it the easiest to grasp. Create yourself a reference by simple Google research on which oils are classified for example as energizing, calming, or any other state of mind or health you are trying to address. To get you started, here is a list of most popular oils and their properties:

Essential Oils By Effect You're After

Energizing - Rosemary, Clary sage, Bergamot, Lemongrass, Eucalyptus, Peppermint, Spearmint, Tea tree, Cypress, Pine, Lemon, Basil, Grapefruit, Ginger.

Calming - Lavender, Geranium, Mandarin, Bergamot, Ylang Ylang, Neroli, Jasmine, Melissa , Palmarosa, Patchouli, Petitgrain, Sandalwood.

Detoxifying - Peppermint, Juniper, Grapefruit, Rosemary, Laurel, Mandarin, Lemon, Patchouli, Hyssop, Helichrysum.

Anti-anxiety

Lavender, Geranium, Roman Chamomile, Marjoram, Sandalwood, Valerian, Bergamot, Jasmine, Black Pepper, Tangerine, Orange, Melissa or Lemon Balm

Blending essential oils that are within the same category usually works well and makes for a mix with complementing qualities.

Similar to a musical scale, essential oils that are quickest to evaporate (usually within 1-2 hours), are called "top notes". Next are the oils that evaporate within 2-4 hours, those are considered "middle notes". The "base notes" are the oils that evaporate the slowest. Some base note oils can take several days to evaporate.

Here are a few examples of popular oils, divided into their oil notes:

Essential Oils By Oil Notes

Top notes - Bergamot, Citronella, Eucalyptus, Grapefruit, Lavender, Lemon, Lemongrass, Lime, Orangge, Peppermint, Spearmint, Tangerine.

Middle notes - Carrot Seed, Chamomile, Cinnamon, Clary Sage, Cypress, Dill, Fennel, Geranium, Jasmine, Marjoram, Neroli, Palmarosa, ROse, Rosemary, Rosewood, Spruce, Tea Tree, Thyme, Ylang Ylang.

Base notes - Angelica Root, Balsam, Cedarwood, Frankincense, Ginger, Helichrysum, Myrrh, Patchouli, Sandalwood, Vanilla, Vetiver.

Blend essential oils with the same oil notes to ensure a blend that keeps smelling and acting consistently over time. Especially if you make a batch, or more than a few drops of a diffuser blend, for your home use.

Start Blending Essential Oils At Home

blending essential oils Now that you've read the three ways to group essential oil types together, basically you're free to let your inner artist shine! With a clear grouping system like this as a base, you can then also choose an essential oil from one category and blend it with an oil from another category. Rather than staying in the same group, this would then allow you to reach combined effects and a "best of both worlds" type of scenario.

Chapter 5

Your Scent Signature

How To Start

It's important to separate yourself from the pack. You need to stand out, and there are a number of ways to accomplish this goal. Many people show off their unique personality through dress, hairstyle, or shoe selection. For something a little more understated, but just as powerful, consider selecting a scent that will immediately identify you to the people you come in contact with everyday. At first, they won't quite know why they're having these powerful, memorable feelings. After all, scent is supposedly the sense most strongly linked to memory. With time, however, they'll come to associate that certain wonderful fragrance with you. Once that connection is made, it won't easily be forgotten.

How can you figure out which scent best matches your style and personality? A large part of the equation is a simple "smell test". Go into any local department store, and try on a number of different perfumes. Pick the one that you like the most, and give it a trial period. Wear it to work, out to the bar, and in other social situations where you'll be in close contact with others. It's wise not to mention that you're trying a new perfume. Let their opinions come to you. That way, you'll know that you're getting honest feedback instead of superfluous compliments.

This first perfume doesn't have to be the signature scent that you're wedded to for eternity. Now it's time to think about the other aspects of the scent. What does it represent? You would be surprised by the subconscious thoughts and ideas that perfumes can trigger in others. A strong perfume will immediately take another person aback, demanding their attention. This could have a mixed result; do you really want to create such a strong impression before you've even had the chance to introduce yourself? Perhaps you'd be better served by something a little less powerful, a scent that flies under the radar until the prey is within reach. Likewise, are you after a more fruity scent, or something that is a bit more masculine?

The scent alone shouldn't be the only consideration for deciding on your signature scent. Perhaps equally important, what is the price tag attached to the bottle? You don't want to get addicted to a perfume that you'll only be able to use sparingly. Consider that your signature perfume is just that: a statement that will make people think of you, and you exclusively. That's why picking something out of your price range is shortsighted. Instead, consider a slightly less expensive option that won't break the bank each month. Choosing your signature perfume should be a fun process, and an expression of exactly what makes you an individual. Remember that you don't have to settle on the first scent that you come across. Take your time, and experiment with different options that best express your personality. As months turn into years, this scent will become a lasting part of your image to the world, and one that people will look to for evidence that you've graced the room with your presence. How you smell is just as important as how you look. In fact sometimes it can be more important. Smell has a way of effecting people in ways looks never could. Have you ever smell a pillow or clothing that had the perfumes of you mate on it? Scents bring back memories and feelings like no other sense.

Create Your Own Perfume

Do you want to make your own signature perfume or cologne scent? Or maybe you're looking for unique homemade gift ideas for friends, family or even co-workers. You can make your very own exciting scents with ingredients from the grocery store. Even nature itself can provide essential ingredients for this ambitious and fun project. Why spend a fortune on perfume or cologne when you can make your own for far less then it would be at stores specializing in this product? Brand name perfume/cologne can cost from $50-200 and much, much more if you shop at a high end retailer. Why spend that much when you can create your own fragrance which is personalized just for you and gives off the fragrance that matches your personality perfectly!

So, know let's go through the process in designing and creating your own personalized perfume/cologne. Know the different notes. Perfumes/colognes are a blend of different levels of scent, also called "notes". When you spray a fragrance on your skin, it moves through these notes in the following order:

Top notes are what you smell first. They are also what disappears first, usually within 10 to 15 minutes.

Middle notes appear as the top notes die off. These are the fragrance's core, determining which family the scent belongs to - for example, oriental, woody, fresh, or floral.

Base notes accentuate and fix the fragrance's middle notes, also known as its theme. They comprise the fragrance's foundation, making the scent last up to 4 or 5 hours on your skin.

Familiarize Yourself With Popular Top Notes.

Popular top notes include basil, bergamot, grapefruit, lavender, lemon, lime, mint, neroli, rosemary, and sweet orange.

Familiarize Yourself With Popular Middle Notes

These include black pepper, cardamom, chamomile, cinnamon, clove, fir needle, jasmine, juniper, lemongrass, neroli, nutmeg, rose, rosewood, and ylang-ylang.

Familiarize Yourself With Popular Base Notes

These include cedarwood, cypress, ginger, patchouli, pine, sandalwood, vanilla, and vetiver.

Know The Ratios : When mixing a fragrance, first add your base notes, then your middle notes, then finally, your top notes. The ideal ratio for blending notes is 30% top notes, 50% middle notes, and 20% base notes. Some people recommend combining a maximum of 3 to 4 dominant notes

Find out what notes your favorite perfumes contain: If you're unsure of how to structure a perfume, have a look at the ingredients of your favorite commercial scents. If you have trouble finding the ingredients or separating them into notes, the Basenotes website is a great resource for breaking down the notes in popular perfumes.

Buy dark glass containers: Many people recommend using dark glass containers because the dark glass helps protect your perfume from light, which can shorten its lifespan. You'll also want to make sure your glass containers haven't previously contained any food items, as any residual scents will transfer to your perfume. The exception to this would be if you actually wanted to use the scent of what was in the glass container before. (Warning: peanut-butter-banana-chocolate perfume might taste better than it smells!)

Buy a carrier oil: A carrier oil is what carries the scents in a particular fragrance on to your skin. These are generally unscented, and are used to dilute concentrated oils and aromatics that can otherwise irritate your skin. Your carrier oil can really be anything. You can even use olive oil if you don't mind the scent. One popular perfumer simmers rose petals in virgin olive oil, then combines it all with vitamin E oil to stabilize it.

Buy the strongest alcohol you can find: A common choice amongst many DIY perfumers is a high-quality, 80- to 100-proof (40% to 50% alc/vol) vodka. Other DIY perfumers favor 190-proof (80% alc/vol) alcohol. Popular choices for 190-proof alcohol include organic neutral grape alcohol and the much cheaper Everclear (a strong American alcohol) which is a grain spirit.

Select your scents: Your perfume can be made out of a wide variety of ingredients. Common aromatics for perfumes include essential oils, flower petals, leaves, and herbs.

Decide on a method: The method for making perfume will vary slightly depending on your materials. Two common aromatics used for perfume are plant materials (flowers, leaves, and herbs) and essential oils; the methods vary for each of these.

Obtain a clean glass container: The type of container isn't as important as the material: just make sure that a) it's clean and b) it's glass. The container also needs to have a tight-fitting lid.

As mentioned before, perfumers generally recommend using dark glass, which can lengthen the fragrance's life by protecting it from light. Avoid using jars that have previously contained food items, even if they've been washed out, as the glass might pass the scent on.

Obtain an odorless oil: Popular choices for use in perfumes include jojoba oil, almond oil, and grape seed oil.

Collect flowers, leaves, or herbs whose scent appeals to you: Be sure to collect plant materials when the scent is strong and the leaves are dry. Letting them air out can leave them limp and with a less effective scent. You may want to collect and dry more plants than you need, just in case you want to add more to strengthen the oil's scent later on.

Remove any unwanted plant materials: If you're using flowers, use only the petals. If you're using leaves or herbs, remove any twigs or other bits that might interfere with the scent.

Bruise the plant materials lightly: This step is optional, but may help to bring out the scent more. You'll just want to lightly press on the plant materials with a wooden spoon.

Pour some oil into the glass container: It need only be a small amount - just enough to properly coat and cover your petals/leaves/herbs.

Add the plant materials to the oil and shut the lid: Ensure that the lid is closed tightly. Let the jar sit in a cool dark place for one to two weeks.

Open, strain and repeat: If the oil doesn't smell as strong as you'd like it to after one to two weeks, you can strain out the old plant materials and add new ones to the scented oil, then store it once more. You can repeat this process for several weeks or even months until the oil has reached the desired strength. Be sure to keep the oil! It's the old plant materials that you want to discard

Preserve your scented oil: Once you're happy with the oil, you can add 1 or 2 drops of a natural preservative such as vitamin E or grapefruit seed extract to your scented oil to help extend its life. If you'd like to turn the oil into a lip balm, you can also add some beeswax to it, melt some beeswax in the microwave, combine it with the perfume, then dump the whole mixture into a container to cool and solidify.

Chapter 6

Perfume Recipes To Start

Almost any mixtures of scents can work, you have to test to know what is your favorites.Making and mixing your own creams, lotions and perfumes can be fun, and not only is it individualized but could also save you some money.

The Basic Perfumes:

1. Old fashioned Eau-de-Cologne

2. 'All alive' perfume

3. Sensual perfume for women

4. Sensual eau de cologne for men

The ideas below are a simple guide for you to get started, but it must be kept in mind that it is easier to add more essential oils to a blend to make the fragrance stronger, than it is to dilute the blend in order to tone the fragrance down. For this reason it is better to rather add too little of an oil, and to top up later if you are looking for a stronger fragrance. One cardinal rule you should always follow, is to write down the recipe, as you are mixing it, as it often happens that a person would prepare a wonderful fragrance, only to find that they cannot remember the quantities or the oils used in the mixture. When mixing your fragrance you should use glass containers, as some plastic containers and instruments do tend to retain fragrance particles. For mixing the blend never use a metal object, but rather use a glass rod.

After you have used your mixing equipment, wash very well with a strong soapy solution, dry, wipe down with alcohol to remove all fragrance traces, wash again, rinse in clean water and dry for next use. For storing your mixed fragrances buy blue or amber glass bottles, and if they have cork stoppers you would need to seal the cork stopper with paraffin wax to prevent oxidation, and if they are equipped with screw tops make sure that the tops have liners.

Essential oils are either added to alcohol or an oil base when making perfumes at home. The alcohol to use is ethanol, but for the sake of ease vodka can be used. It is best to buy a high quality 100% proof vodka since it has virtually no smell.

The oil base that can be used is jojoba oil which is really a liquid wax. Jojoba has excellent keeping properties and does not have a very heavy odor of its own.

The percentage of essential oil used in perfumes is high, and to prevent any allergic reaction, remember to do a skin patch test if you have never used a particular oil, and also look at our page on essential oil safety by clicking here.

When blending your perfume or eau de toilette or cologne start with the base (alcohol/vodka or oil base depending on what you are making) and add the oils drop by drop.

The classification of perfume, eau de toilette and eau de cologne is based on the strength of the fragrance it contains and the percentages of essences used.

For a perfume you will use around 15% essential oil, whilst for a lighter eau de toilette you will use about 4 - 8% essential oil and a yet lighter eau de cologne 1 - 5%.

If you want to work out your percentages, you can work on the premise that 1 ml is 20 drops. To work out your percentages convert the total of the oil used as well as the base - be that the alcohol/vodka or jojoba oil - to drops.

If your total drops are, let's say 58 drops, and your base 240 ml (240 x 20 = 4,800 drops) divide the amount of drops by the amount of drops in the base. Using the above example you will get a result of 0.012 = 1.2% concentrate of oil in the mixture.

Some of the recipes state that you should mix the blend, bottle, cap and leave for x amount of days. This is to give the fragrance time to settle and to achieve a more rounded fragrance.

Old Fashioned Eau-De-Cologne

- ✓ 16 drops bergamot
- ✓ 15 drops petitgrain
- ✓ 2 drops orange
- ✓ 15 drops lemon
- ✓ 5 drops lavender
- ✓ 5 drops neroli
- ✓ 10 ml orange flower water
- ✓ 230 ml alcohol/vodka

Place the alcohol/vodka base into your glass mixing container, add the oils in the order listed and mix well. Bottle, cap and leave the mixture for 4 days and then add the orange flower water and re-cap. Leave the mixture for at least two weeks, giving the bottle a gentle shake every day.

'All Alive' Perfume

- ✓ 4 drops sweet orange
- ✓ 10 drops lemon
- ✓ 6 drops tangerine
- ✓ 8 drops frankincense
- ✓ 5 drops neroli
- ✓ 1 drop myrrh
- ✓ 10 ml alcohol/vodka or
- ✓ 10 ml jojoba oil for a oil based perfume.

Place the base into your mixing container and add the ingredients in the order listed and mix. Bottle and use. You can reduce the base, but do note your concentration will then exceed 15%.

Sensual Perfume For Women

- ✓ 5 drops coriander

- ✓ 6 drops bergamot

- ✓ 4 drops neroli

- ✓ 1 drops jasmine blend

- ✓ 3 drops rose blend

- ✓ 10 ml jojoba oil

Place oil base in mixing container, add oils in the order listed and mix. Bottle, cap and leave one week before using.

Sensual eau de cologne for men

- ✓ 10 drops lavender

- ✓ 20 drops coriander

- ✓ 22 drops sandalwood

- ✓ 23 drops cedarwood

- ✓ 5 drop frankincense

- ✓ 100 ml alcohol/vodka

Place the alcohol/vodka mixture into your mixing bowl, add the oils in the order given and mix well.

The above is my humble contribution to fragrance mixing and is really basic. Your personal taste will determine what you like.

Chapter 7

Your Perfume Loves You

When you invest in yourself you will always get rewarded. All your system will thank you and you will get compliments from your surroundings.

Did you know certain scents can affect your perception of time? Coffee enhances and heightens your awareness of time and the scent of jasmine increases your reaction time. Discover how these scents that you smell daily can affect your emotions.

According to some studies, yes, fragrance can both affect and change your mood. Not only does fragrance affect mood, but it can actually enhance work performance and behavior in various ways. It almost seems magical, but according to science, the fragrance is not working on "us." We work on the fragrance through life experiences with them.

This is based on "associative learning." Associative learning is the process of items or events linking to a person's individual past experiences. Certain fragrances may trigger certain feelings and emotions for different people. What might bring peace and serenity to some, many not be the same for others.

Perfumes Affect The Mood

Many perfumes and fragrances offer a sort of aromatherapy quality and effect, and can easily work to alter the mood. Knowing that fragrances have this power to alter and affect mood, perfume companies and fragrance companies work diligently in creating new fragrances that will offer positive mood change benefits.

Some of the positive mood change benefits that you can expect to find from a perfume with aromatherapy qualities include:

- ✓ Increased alertness

- ✓ Invigoration

- ✓ Uplifting mood

- ✓ Relaxation

- ✓ Feeling motivated

How Do I Know Which Fragrance To Choose From?

By trying them out and testing them. Breathe in the scents of various perfumes and fragrances, then go by your own personal instincts as to which fragrance you think will not only make you smell lovely but that might also offer some added aromatherapy benefits. You should learn which scents bring about the mood or feeling that you're looking for.

Aromatherapy is sometimes used as an alternative medicine process to enhance one's mood and overall general well-being by incorporating natural and essential oils from various sources such as flowers and stems, leaves and bark, as well as other plant parts.

Some popular perfumes with aromatherapy and mood enhancing qualities include: Lavender Frankincense Perfume – Botanical Perfume, Victoria's Secret Fantasies Love Spell Fragrance Mist, Viva La Juicy by Couture, Eternity by Calvin Klein, Vera Wang Princess by Vera Wang, Cool Water by Zino Davidoff and many more.

Why You Should Choose Perfume When You're In A Good Mood Vs. A Bad Mood

Did you know that the mood you're in will greatly affect your ability to choose the right perfume while perfume shopping? It can and that is because your mood affect's your body's PH balance. When you're in a good mood, your body is balanced and your olfactory sensory system (your sense of smell) is at its peak. But when you're in a bad mood, the effects of stress and other factors can inhibit your olfactory system. So you'll want to perfume shop when stress levels are low and you're in high-spirits.

Aromatherapy Affects Emotions

Fragrances grab your attention. Consider how you feel when you smell the enticing aroma of freshly baked brownies or bread, the appealing scent of coffee brewing in the morning, or the scent of certain perfumes and colognes that suddenly stir up memories of the past. From these examples it is easy to see that aromatherapy really does affect our emotions. Aromas and fragrances affect us in a way that is both primitive and alluring. Aromatherapy affects emotions in many different ways. Aromatherapy can be used to help us relax, to provide mental clarity, to help cope with emotional conflicts, and to energize us physically, emotionally or mentally.

When we smell something, information is sent to specific parts of our brain that influences memory, basic emotions, learning, etc. Fragrances can be used to influence people and how they feel about themselves, and even how they interact with each other. With this in mind, you can incorporate fragrances and scents into your everyday life to improve the way you feel about and respond to life. And you can even covertly influence those around you. Aromatherapy is often accomplished through the use of essential oils which are a true concentrated essence extracted from a plant. Essential oils are very potent, and much can be accomplished through the use of just a few drops.

Below is a brief list of fragrances and their effects on emotions. Many of these fragrances have been used for centuries getting these same results.

Scents to Relieve Anger: Chamomile, Jasmine, Patchouli, Rose and Ylang-ylang.

Scents to Relieve Anxiety: Bergamot, Cedarwood, Cypress, Frankincense, Hyssop, Lavender, Marjoram, Myrrh, Neroli, Orange, Peach, Rose, Rose Geranium and Violet Leaf.

Scents to Increase Confidence: Frankincense, Jasmine, Patchouli and Sandalwood.

Scents to Ease Depression: Bergamot, Clary Sage, Grapefruit, Jasmine, Lavender, Lemon, Lemon Balm, Lemon Verbena, Neroli, Orange, Petitgrain, Rose Geranium, Sandalwood, Tangerine and Ylang-ylang.

Scents to Improve Memory: Bay Laurel, Jasmine, Lavender, Lemon and Rosemary.

Scents to Ease Sorrow: Clary Sage, Cypress, Fir, Marjoram, Rosemary and Sage.

Scents Used as Aphrodisiacs: Jasmine, Rose, Sandalwood, Vanilla and Ylang-ylang.

Scents to Invigorate and Overcome Fatigue: Angelica, Benzoin, Camphor, Cardamom, Cinnamon, Clove Basil, Cypress, Eucalyptus, Fennel, Lemon, Peppermint, Pine, Sage and Spiced Apple.

Scents to Deal with Stress, Nervous Tension and Insomnia: Bergamot, Chamomile, Cinnamon, Cloves, Frankincense, Lavender, Lemon, Marjoram, Myrrh, Neroli, Nutmeg, Orange, Petitgrain, Rose, Sandalwood, Sweet Melissa, Valerian, Vanilla, Violet, and Ylang-ylang.

Scents to Calm Irritability: Chamomile, Neroli, Rose, and Rose Geranium.

CONCLUSION

There are so many wonderful scents and fragrances to choose from that can both inspire and alter mood, which makes it all the more fun for perfume lovers everywhere to experiment with and add to their perfume collections.

In contrast, alcohol based perfumes can evaporate more quickly from the body due to the high percentage of alcohol in the mixture. They are certainly more diffusive than oil based perfume and permeate the wearers surrounding unlike oil based perfumes that are much more intimate to wear. No matter what type of base used in a perfume, the result can be an outstanding one if the right steps to perfume making are properly followed.

Creating one's very own perfume is a personal thing, it's not a one size fits all selection process to choose what fragrant essences should go in the blend. The process is very flexible and there are many varieties of perfume classifications to appeal to different tastes. Some perfumes are specifically designed for men or women, while others can appeal to both sexes. Either way, perfumes are personal reflection of the wearers taste. So, if you are interested in making perfumes for personal use, it's all about you and how you like to smell.

Thank you very much for reading the book. If you loved the book, I would appreciate it if you can write a review of the book for me. If you have any question about the book feel free to contact me at orilaor@outlook.com.

For 20$ Coupon for www.laorcare.com were you can find all the professional products to clear your Pigmentation, send the word: PERFECTION to my mail.

With sincere love Ori Laor